Ehlers Danlos Syndrome:
What Causes the Pain?

Dr. Christopher Maloney, N.D.

ISBN: 1512376620
ISBN-13: 978-1512376623

DEDICATION

To those that suffer, that they might find relief.

CONTENTS

ACKNOWLEDGMENTS

I thank my family, my teachers, and the worldwide community of researchers who selflessly provide us all with knowledge.

DISCLAIMER

The following is a discussion about Ehlers-Danlos Syndrome, also called Joint Hypermobility Syndrome. It is meant to increase your knowledge of the Syndrome, not to take the place of medical consultation. Please discuss the information provided with your physician.

1

WHAT IS JOINT HYPERMOBILITY SYNDROME?

Because Joint Hypermobility Syndrome encompasses a range of different Syndromes, we will talk mostly about it as the older Ehlers-Danlos Syndrome (EDS) even though the names are becoming interchangeable:

Experts now think Joint Hypermobility is likely the most common connective tissue disease in the world.[i] As the number of types of hypermobility disorders has been growing in the U.S., the NIH has produced an entire online book to help patients and doctors distinguish between the subtypes of the syndromes.[ii]

Because the basic criteria of these Syndromes may not be familiar to many readers, here are the basic guidelines (adapted from the Hypermobility Syndromes Association[iii]) for determining if you have either illness.

The first thing you need to do is a little physical movement. This will help you figure out if you have a Hypermobility Syndrome by determining your Beighton Score.

The **Beighton score** is calculated as follows:
- One point if while standing forward bending you can place palms on the ground with legs straight
- One point for each elbow that bends backwards
- One point for each knee that bends backwards
- One point for each thumb that touches the forearm when bent backwards
- One point for each little finger that bends backwards beyond 90 degrees.
  What is your Beighton score?

Major Criteria of Joint Hypermobility Syndrome.

➢ A **Beighton score** of 4/9 or greater (either currently or historically)
➢ And/Or Joint Pain for longer than 3 months in 4 or more joints

Minor Criteria

- A Beighton score of 1, 2 or 3/9 (0, 1, 2 or 3 if aged 50+)
- And/Or joint pain (> 3 months) in one to three joints or back pain (> 3 months), with bone spurring.
- Dislocation/subluxation (do your joints pop out of place or partially out of place) in more than one joint, or in one joint on more than one occasion.
- Soft tissue chronic swelling > 3 months.
- Marfanoid appearance (tall, slim, arms longer than height, legs longer than torso, long slim fingers).

- Abnormal skin: tear marks, overly flexible, thin, easily scarred.
- Eye signs: drooping eyelids or shortsighted or oddly slanted.
- Varicose veins/hernias/prolapses.

Another quick tool to use is the hypermobility questionnaire. An answer of 'Yes' to 2 or more of the questions gives a very high prediction of the presence of hypermobility. Again, like the Beighton score, this makes it more likely but does not mean that the person absolutely has a Hypermobility Syndrome.

Here are the hypermobility questionnaire questions:

1. Can you now (or could you ever) place your hands flat on the floor without bending your knees?
2. Can you now (or could you ever) bend your thumb to touch your forearm?
3. As a child did you amuse your friends by contorting your body into strange shapes OR could you do the splits?
4. As a child or teenager did your shoulder or kneecap dislocate on more than one occasion?
5. Do you consider yourself double-jointed?

The difficulty in assessing an illness based on physical symptoms is that many people may meet some of the criteria but not others. So while the awareness of joint hypermobility is expanding some experts think that the high numbers cannot be trusted because only some of the included patients truly have the syndrome.

Even if the numbers are exaggerated, they are truly stunning. Joint hypermobility was found in one in four people, only about one in ten men but almost one in three women. People with joint hypermobility weren't more likely to get injured but were more likely to have sprains, back pain, and stress fractures.[iv]

The number of individuals with hypermobility is much higher in some professions. In a group of ballet dancers the majority had joint hypermobility. Teachers of ballet were three times as likely as their students to have joint hypermobility.[v] In patients at rheumatology or physical therapy clinics the chances of finding joint hypermobility is much higher than in the general population and is even higher if the patients are minorities.[vi]

Given the extent to which Joint Hypermobility Syndrome/EDS causes pain and suffering to a substantial portion of the population, almost nothing is known about it and few treatments are available. Let's explore why.

2
GENETICS

My patient can touch her toes to the back of her head at sixty. It's not something she thinks about, because she's always been able to do it. What she's seeing me about is pain. Sometimes, she hurts so much that even narcotics cannot fully relieve the pain. Medicinal marijuana helps her, but she's eating far more because sometimes nothing helps.

In the past my patient would be diagnosed with Ehlers-Danlos Syndrome (EDS), but now that syndrome is being slowly changed over to a wider group of diseases that fall under Joint Hypermobility Syndrome. So now instead of having a firm diagnosis she's not even sure what to say she has to new doctors.

Even when it was just EDS, there were already eight subtypes of EDS. Some of them were far more lethal than others, so patients would receive the diagnosis and panic unnecessarily.

To avoid confusion, I will talk about joint hypermobility using the shorthand of EDS. Since much of this book is speculative, rather than proven, take everything I say with a large grain of salt (or potassium if you're trying to cut down).

EDS is a genetic disease. It is passed from parent to child, and only occasionally occurs without parental involvement (a genetic mutation). Family members sharing the same genes can have variations of the Syndrome.

Because it is classified as a genetic disease, the standard treatments for Ehlers-Danlos are all supportive, designed to help manage and monitor the disease rather than cure it. Once diagnosed, patients get monitored and given what medical support can be given. Usually this includes heart and blood vessel monitoring as these areas need rapid repair if they begin to fail. Treatment may also include various types of pain relief, including various narcotic agents to try and help relieve daily suffering.

But because of its assumed genetic nature, very little serious research is being done on the causes and possible treatments of Ehlers-Danlos Syndrome. A medical search for EDS turns up about three thousand articles, which is approximately the same number that cover foot bunions. For comparison, an illness like osteoporosis (bone loss) has seventy thousand articles. So while there is a little information, most researchers have closed the book on EDS. We have the cause: genetics. We have the treatments: surgery and pain support. So this should be a very short book and end here.

But it doesn't end because genetics do not fully explain EDS. Based on the limited research done so far, we do not fully understand the cause. Genetic testing is done on all family members during an EDS investigation. Patients with extreme symptoms and family members with no symptoms BOTH show the genetic mutations in collagen formation that indicates EDS. So the genetic mutations do not impact the Beighton score and they do not have anything to do with the level of pain experienced by the individuals.

Family members who have no symptoms can also display the same genetic tendencies toward malformation and hyperextension as patients writhing in agony. They have the same genetics and some of the same flexibility without presenting with pain symptoms. So the pain experienced by an individual with EDS may not be simply genetic in origin.

The idea that the pain of EDS is not caused by the genetic disease can be difficult to believe. Let me discuss one of the studies I'm using.[vii]

Researchers tracked twenty-seven different patients with EDS born into seventeen different, unrelated families. Over three years, they collected skin biopsies from all the twenty-seven EDS patients and sixty-four of their relatives.

The skin biopsies showed classic tissue changes in all the patients diagnosed with either EDS or Joint Hypermobility Syndrome. But only twenty-six of their relatives had normal skin. The others, without symptoms, had the same tissue changes as those who had been diagnosed.

Given the same genetics, researchers were surprised that some family members did not have disease symptoms. They speculated that perhaps those family members had "outgrown" their EDS. Since EDS symptoms typically show up later in life and worsen, this seems unlikely.

Other researchers testing families with clear genetic transfer of joint hypermobility found Beighton scores between 9 and 2. They noted how common joint hypermobility is, how it has a genetic component, but how often it is "benign" and causes no symptoms.[viii] Genetics alone do not determine pain for an EDS patient.

These results show genetics only explain part of the Syndrome. If we do not yet have the full cause, is it possible that we may not have exhausted all possible treatments for the condition?

3
PAIN ONSET

The model given to my patient for the cause of her pain from her EDS is relatively simple. Her body's hypermobile joints have repeatedly over-extended over time and have become loose enough to cause her pain.

Based on that model, we would expect a person with EDS to experience pain directly as a result of over-using any joint. They would be more prone to arthritis pain from overuse, and experience more pain if they used already painful joints.

We would further expect that the pain of EDS sufferers would occur at any age, because the pain is due to overuse. A young runner with EDS would experience pain based on how much she runs. In contrast, a sedentary couch potato lifestyle would be the best way for EDS patients to stay relatively pain free for most of their lives. No strain, no pain.

So when does the pain of EDS occur? We don't have a clear answer. As mentioned in the last chapter, many individuals with the EDS genetic picture never develop symptoms. So it's difficult to determine when a pain comes on due to the disease process.

The worst form of EDS, type III, should show up sooner than other types based on the overuse model. Type III EDS is known for severe heart and heart vessel involvement. The heart and blood vessels are constantly being pushed to overextend. But researchers warn that less than one in five patients with the worst kind of type III EDS will have any symptoms before they show up at the emergency room with serious heart issues, sometimes with arteries rupturing without warning.[ix]

If even the worst form of EDS can remain a "stealth" syndrome and only manifest suddenly with severe complications, then we have no clear indication of when or even if pain will manifest for a patient with EDS.

But surely EDS sufferers can predict pain worsening as a result of overuse, and easing based on resting periods? Doesn't that show their pain comes from overuse? Yes, most EDS patients with pain of any age are improved with rest after overuse. But when they are children EDS patients do not typically experience more pain than their peers from overuse and many EDS children outperform their peers physically.[x] As they get older, researchers have tracked EDS diagnosed children with pain alongside those EDS children who do not develop pain symptoms. The EDS children with pain become more flexible than other EDS children, their skin stretched more, and they urinated out far more tissue breakdown wastes when compared to EDS children who did not develop symptoms. Both sets of children start with the genetic and physical diagnosis of EDS, yet only part of that genetic group goes on to develop pain.[xi] Some other systemic change, not simple overuse, is causing EDS patients to descend down the pathway to chronic pain.

4
CURRENT PAIN MODEL ISSUES

For patients with EDS, the current pain model is remarkably simple. Hyper-extended joints and tissues wear down, and result in pain. In the worst case scenario, internal vessels wear down and need surgical repair. But beyond surgery, patients are requested to move as little as possible. It all makes very good sense until you look closer.

The pain model does explain many symptoms that commonly occur with EDS patients. Sprains are very common for EDS patients, and one in ten EDS patients has had dislocation of joints. Bruising happens easily. Almost half of EDS patients have difficulty with handwriting, and most had difficulty with physical activities. Due to physical symptoms many EDS sufferers miss significant amounts of schooling.

But other common EDS symptoms are less well explained by the hyperextension model of pain. Urinary tract infections are common. So are speech and learning disabilities. Dyslexia (reversing words) and dyspraxia (poor coordination) indicates that there is a brain effect to this illness that cannot be explained by the overuse of joints. Despite having loose joints, boys with EDS have five times as much constipation, while girls have more urinary incontinence.[xii]

The extent of the expansion of other symptoms in EDS beyond joint pain has caused a recent critique of EDS being defined as a hypermobility disorder. While it is often discovered using hypermobility as a marker, the symptoms of EDS have expanded beyond joints into practically all major body systems and organs.[xiii]

But, as long as all these new symptoms are caused by genetics, the only treatment continues to be supportive care. Yes, we may expand our diagnostic net to include other body systems besides the joints, but that information just gets put in the chart. If genetic changes cause all EDS symptoms we aren't going to be looking for a cure. We're just looking to manage the illness over the patient's lifetime.

No one is doing anything wrong by not doing more. Researchers commonly overlook a disease that is considered genetic because in many, many cases nothing more can be done. Many of our current birth defects are caused by errors in genetic material, and these typically cause difficulty for patients throughout their lifetimes. While there are a few experimental genetic treatments, we've discovered nothing that will permanently correct the defect. Once a disease has been classified as genetic, it falls into the same category as an amputation. You do what you can to support a normal life, but you don't go looking for another cause.

5
CURRENT TREATMENT

Given the genetic nature of EDS within the current model, there are no curative treatments. The only treatment that has any noticeable effect is surgery. So are EDS patients regularly scheduled for repairing surgeries? Do they regularly get tendons tightened? No.

Based on the available research, EDS patients make horrible surgical candidates. Anything invasive should be avoided unless an EDS patient could die. An EDS patient's skin tissue tends to be soft, and that also includes inner tissues like intestines and other organs. A surgeon trying to cut into an EDS patient will have easy going, but the nightmare starts when trying to sew an EDS patient closed. The two edges of the wound are slippery and difficult to align properly. Using a needle and suture on such soft tissue causes easy tearing. After several notable cases of massive bleeding during operations which resulted in massive scarring inside the abdomen or the death of the patients, surgeons have been warned away from doing any surgery that can be avoided.[xiv]

In some cases surgeons may not intervene surgically specifically because a patient has an EDS diagnosis. In a case of massive abdominal bleeding in an EDS patient, the patient was not treated surgically. The surgeon was aware of other reports of surgery resulting in death of the patient so did not intervene and the patient survived. Because of the EDS diagnosis, the surgeon rightly did not consider an abdomen full of blood to be a surgical emergency.[xv]

If surgery is rarely an option unless facing death, surely we at least have a great deal of research on pain management for EDS patients? Not really. We don't even have any idea how much pain they experience. In the latest review of EDS in 2012, there wasn't an agreed-upon international measure of EDS pain.[xvi] If you can't measure it, how can you know how well you are controlling it?

It's the extent and variety of EDS pain that defies a single measure. Sure, a patient experiences joint and muscle pain. But also nerve pain, pelvic pain, abdominal pain, and muscle weakness. Add in headache, fatigue, digestive issues, and unrefreshing sleep, and you get a sense that the symptoms of EDS overlap with many other conditions that a patient may have.

The drugs used for EDS patients also mostly overlap with drugs used for arthritis, rheumatoid arthritis, or chronic pain generally. But EDS patients may not experience the expected relief from these pain medications because the one of the symptoms of EDS can include a resistance to anesthetic agents.[xvii]

A study of the current treatment of EDS sufferers found that over 90% of EDS patients take pain medications. And, despite the dangers, 70% of EDS patients have had surgery.

Yet only half of EDS patients are involved in physical therapy. Patients who had massage, learned exercises, and had electrical stimulation found great relief. But physical therapy involves movement, and many doctors consider any movement to be harmful.

Only about a third of EDS patients undergoing surgery had good results, while twice as many reported feeling better after physical therapy.[xviii] Given the risk of surgery, more physical therapy should be the norm. But it flies in the face of the widely held belief that EDS patients shouldn't overdo it. No strain, no pain. If only that worked. Strengthening the system around torn joints seems to work better.

6
AN ALTERNATIVE MODEL

What if the genetics and the loose joints of EDS weren't the cause of pain for patients? Remember the studies that failed to find a consistent connection between genetics and pain. What if hypermobility is also not the determining factor for EDS pain? Let's take a moment to look at what this might mean. In a world where genetics and hypermobility did not cause pain, another factor, let's call it Factor X, would be involved.

It's worthwhile thinking about Factor X affecting EDS patients because it might be resolvable. Just avoid Factor X, and you can keep your EDS genes without the pain. Unlike the genetic/hypermobility model, the idea of another disturbing factor leads to a host of possibilities for both treatment and management.

Individuals with the genetic makeup of EDS would be vulnerable to this Factor X, whether it was infectious, autoimmune, or environmental. Only when this Factor X was activated would the genetic predisposition of EDS sufferers be activated and cause pain. In other words, what if it takes genetics AND hypermobility AND something else (Factor X) to cause EDS pain.

Certainly adding another factor would explain the variation in presentation among EDS sufferers. Family members who share the genetic makeup but who don't have an activating Factor X would experience no symptoms until the factor affected them as well.

Following this exploration, we might ask ourselves what the nature of this Factor X might be. In medicine we have a number of different general causes of diseases. They include infections, environmental causes, autoimmune reactions, and hormonal imbalances.

So what sort of Factor X are we looking for? And how would we go about teasing out that kind of trigger from what little we know about EDS patients?

If Factor X were infectious or environmental, it might spread among susceptible individuals. You could catch EDS from your family, or get it from drinking water with Factor X in it. It might not be that contagious, only mildly like Leprosy, so that you must have a lot of intimate contact with a person to get it and it wouldn't spread to strangers through a handshake.

If Factor X were environmental, something in our air and water, it wouldn't be as common in specific families and nowhere else. Even if your family is particularly sensitive to something in the water, somewhere in the world there are people who are consuming such massive quantities of this EDS causing toxin that some of them would have symptoms. Instead, we have EDS limited to genetic families. So it's not as likely to be an environmental trigger. We cannot ignore that some families may simply be more susceptible to something in their environment, but we currently have no evidence that a particular environment encourages EDS.

If we look for any possible infectious Factor X for EDS, we simply have no information. Although researchers acknowledge the changeable presentation of the symptoms over time, they have no explanation for why this week an EDS patient is improving and next week she is in agony. We are still consumed by the process of categorizing different types of EDS based on genetic abnormalities. No one is seriously looking for any other cause. But we would expect that family members in close proximity for long periods would be more likely to get EDS compared to family that was more distant. Hopefully researchers would have noticed that situation, as well as noting that some of those in close contact with EDS patients came down with EDS even though they weren't genetically related. Since we have no evidence for an infectious cause, we should move on for now.

The most obvious Factor X, closely related to genetics, would be an autoimmune reaction. Autoimmune reactions (poison oak, seafood allergies, etc.) respond to steroids and immune suppressing chemotherapy drugs in the conventional medical model. So one of the ways we could find out if Factor X is autoimmune is by looking for studies on EDS patients' pain control using steroids or immune suppressing chemotherapy. If the pain is caused by an immune reaction, blocking the immune system with steroids or other drugs should lessen the pain.

Steroids have not been used in the treatment of EDS, at least nothing has been reported in the literature. Neither have any chemotherapeutic agents. So, strangely, we can't tell if they would be effective for the pain of EDS.

We do have some basic information about autoimmune reactions and EDS. EDS patients do better with rest. In comparison, most autoimmune conditions like rheumatoid arthritis worsen from rest. With autoimmune arthritis, leaving a joint in one position during sleep often promotes increased pain and stiffness.[xix] But EDS patients commonly experience relief from sleep. So EDS is less likely to be autoimmune.

Until more research is done on the other possibilities, the only research we have that might be useful documents the rapid decline of EDS patients. An autoimmune patient would tend to swell up more and more during her decline, while an infected patient would get sicker and sicker. That's not what we see.

The reports of EDS patients in crisis are based on severe internal breakdowns which require surgery to save the EDS patients' life. In the case of EDS type IV, which affects internal organs and can lead to rupture, the case histories of patients in crisis stretch from a five-year-old girl up to a forty-year-old woman. No discussion is given as to why the intestinal ruptures occur when they do. Surely a child should have less chance of rupturing than an adult?

Instead, the surgeons note that their efforts are often in vain. Once a patient with EDS type IV starts rupturing their bowel, they keep doing it. The high rate of return patients has made the surgeons unwilling to do multiple surgeries. Instead, they leave the patients with a colostomy. A colostomy is when the bowel is bypassed and you literally get to poop in a plastic bag attached to your belly for the rest of your life. It beats dying, even if you have to do it at a very young age.[xx]

In this situation, because the intestines are considered optional, it is simply easier to take them all out once they begin to rupture. But what causes the initial rupture, and why does it recur once it has begun?

While the initial cause eludes us, we have a clue as to why the intestinal ruptures would recur. After surgery, a number of reports talk about multiple adhesions of scar tissue. EDS patients not only have hypermobility, they also have abnormal scarring, perhaps as part of the same collagen tissue imbalance.

Perhaps the EDS tendency toward internal scarring is something like the model of keloid-forming patients. Patients who form keloids have a hyper-response to trauma, causing their skin to go wild and form far more scar tissue than is necessary to heal the wound. In the case of EDS patients the internal scarring could be so wide spread it makes the intestines much more prone to tearing after an initial surgery. In other words, it is the scarring, not the hypermobility, that leads to the recurrent trauma in type IV patients.

Expanding on that same model, is it possible that the process of tissue breakdown leading to excess scarring is a cause of problems in other parts of EDS patients' bodies?

During studies of tissue tearing in healthy skin, all forms of repair are used. The body uses collagen, a thick filler material, to knit together a wound. Different types of collagen have different names (elastin, helical, etc.), but all of them are engaged during healthy tissue repair.[xxi]

EDS patients have problems with maintaining all the types of healthy collagen. At some point in the wound healing process an EDS patient's tissue breaks down much more quickly than a person with all tissue collagen types intact. But even the compromised collagen of an EDS patient may be able to last for decades or a lifetime without rupture. Something must change in the tissue that not only allows the complete breakdown, but also sets up scar formation leading to further tearing.

What could do that in the body? Let's go back to the beginning. Healthy children without EDS are more flexible on average than adults. Most become less flexible over time unless they take an active interest in remaining flexible.

In a study of scarring researchers found that adults scar easily, but wounds on embryos heal perfectly with no scars. So researchers isolated out the factors found in embryos and tried injecting them into adults. Those adults experienced scar-free healing as long as they had those factors injected.[xxii] Could this embryonic mix reverse the scarring in EDS patients as well? And could its lack be causing the over-scarring that EDS patients experience?

The loss of the factors within the body that prevent scarring may take place slowly over time, or may take place quite quickly. If scarring were to be the cause, not only of internal rupture, but also of chronic pain, then that would explain the variation in both onset of symptoms and the worsening of symptoms once the scarring has begun.

Just as the internal organs scar and rescar, the body's peripheral muscles can tear and retear. With each tear comes a new overly large scar, leading to a tighter muscle or ligament surrounded by more mobile, hyperextending tissue. As the injured area continues to be reinjured, it continues to tighten. The result is both chronic pain and immobility in that area. Once one area is immobile, other body areas must compensate, making them more prone to injury. As the number of injured areas mounts, the scarring worsens. A patient is left with both chronic pain and partial immobility, with only a gradual descent into more pain possible.

Although we know relatively little about the possible factors causing the manifestation of EDS symptoms in genetically susceptible individuals, we can look for different solutions if we redirect our attention away from the hypermobility of EDS to think about a scarring/inflammatory model. Using this model, it is not the hypermobility of the patient that causes pain, but the scarring of injured tissues. Thinking about EDS pain as a result of scarring and inflammation has far reaching consequences in terms of treatment.

7
POSSIBLE TREATMENT

When looking at possible treatment for EDS from a point of view of scarring rather than hypermobility, a shift needs to take place in our viewpoint. No longer would it be ideal to surgically tighten joints or tissues, it will just make matters worse. If you recall the surgeon's advice to avoid surgery if at all possible, we should add that any surgery should be as non-invasive as possible. Do not attempt to shorten anything, leave it as long and loose as possible.

Currently EDS patients are placed in a variety of braces and told to isolate and lock down joints. But those who had regular physical therapy including massage and stretching had better outcomes. The gentle lengthening of scar tissue is absolutely essential for continued motion. Bracing and isolating joints only adds to tightening and won't work long term unless a patient can hold that joint immobile for the rest of her life.

If EDS pain is caused by scar tissue, then suddenly the whole range of treatments commonly used for scarring become available. Anything that can be used to break down scarring should be considered, and trials can begin. In simplest terms, patients with EDS should exhaust all treatments related to scarring before resigning themselves to a life of chronic pain.

In the last chapter we looked at a study of scarring where the researchers had actually isolated factors that decreased scarring. If scarring is the cause of chronic pain in EDS patients, then a trial of scar suppression would make sense.

Unfortunately the research study was done on animals, and it is unlikely that we will have human trials that allow researchers to inject humans with the combination they found worked so well. In a world where EDS was considered treatable, such research would take place. But we live in a world that considers

EDS both genetic and untreatable. So it is unlikely we'll see any human trials in this area unless they are done for cosmetic scar reduction in burn victims or cosmetic surgical patients.

While we wait for those trials to take place, there may be something we can take from the scar research. Researchers isolated out one of the many factors that helped animals live scar-free, a chemical called TGFβ3. Giving that chemical alone greatly reduced the scarring and restored the collagen.[xxiii]

So where can we get some of this chemical? A relatively common compound increased the scar suppression chemical TGFβ3 in animals.[xxiv] It's a variation on tryptophan, an amino acid. Tryptophan is popularly known as an antidepressant because of its ability to generate serotonin. Serotonin is the brain chemical that is also increased by common antidepressants like Prozac. Because of past contamination of tryptophan many stores carry it as 5HTP, or 5 hydroxy-tryptophan. It is possible that taking tryptophan could increase the anti-scarring TGFβ3 in humans. If that occurred, and if the pain is caused by scarring, then it is possible that the pain would decrease.

Another route would be to seek a prescription form of a similar compound. A tryptophan (5-HT, again slightly different) increasing drug is marketed for patients with Irritable Bowel Syndrome under the brand name Tegaserod. But most patients will need to consult with their doctors about adding an over-the-counter supplement.

But what could we expect for side effects from tryptophan? For those schooled in alternatives, tryptophan (5-HTP) is commonly given for depression and anxiety, something that hypermobile children experience at a higher rate than the general population.[xxv] 5-HTP is relatively safe, but may interact with antidepressants. Patients trying to lose weight have used up to 900 mg, but nausea can be a common side effect at lower doses.

In looking at supplementation, a number of other common supplements could be used, including: calcium, carnitine, coenzyme Q(10), glucosamine, magnesium, methyl sulphonyl methane, pycnogenol, silica, vitamin C, and vitamin K.[xxvi] To these we add all muscle relaxants, muscle warmers (essential oils), and a host of supportive nutrients. Unfortunately, we don't have any studies on humans to clarify which of these compounds may be the most useful.

As we expand our search for treatments, new hyped treatments like Sirtuin research (resveratrol or red wine extract) might seem attractive because it works for everything. But the goal is to find substances that specifically have been shown to help resolve scar tissue. There are more than enough of those to occupy trials for a number of years.

One specific area that has promise is the use of enzymes that are known to break down scar tissue. In animal studies of Papain (an enzyme found in papayas) the scars treated were significantly decreased compared with the control group. Papain is readily available in most grocery stores as a digestive enzyme. Since the animal dosage was directly applied to the scar, any trial of papain or similar enzyme orally would involve very large doses.

From a physical therapy standpoint, anything strenuous that will tear tissue is to be avoided. But treatment with something like an ultrasound machine, which is known to break down fibrotic tissue, should be considered. And a range of massage techniques that separate and lengthen muscle fibers without tearing them should be on the treatment options. Currently physical therapists are limited by doctor's prescriptions as to what treatments they can do. In this case an independent consultation with a physical therapist might be in order to get the full range of his or her expertise regarding an individual case.

If a doctor were wanting to explore both scar prevention and a possible infectious cause, then Doxycycline has been shown to not only kill bacteria, but also slows collagen degradation.[xxvii] It is that sort of dual action in drugs that patients with EDS should be aware of. In general terms a wet, incubator-like microenvironment provides the fastest healing with the least scarring of human tissue.[xxviii] Keep bandages and gauze on any wound until it has completely healed to minimize the chance of scarring.

So drugs that decrease fluids (like many hypertension medications) would also dehydrate tisse and possibly increase scar formation. Taking in compounds like caffeine will also increase urination and possible dehydration. Looking at one's whole medical picture from a point of view of avoiding scarring may lead to insights that prevent worse future pain.

8
FACTOR X?

In the last decade we've seen an explosion in research on a relatively minor hormone called relaxin that might apply to EDS. While we don't know for certain, it might just be that critical Factor X that creates or modifies pain in EDS patients.

Relaxin has been known for decades as a hormone necessary for a successful pregnancy. It allows the fibers of muscles and ligaments in a pregnant woman to relax and allow the growth of the child. The highest levels of relaxin were seen in the first three months of pregnancy, and the only purpose relaxin was thought to have served in men was increasing sperm motility.

But that perspective on relaxin has changed. In a recent study of healthy non-pregnant volunteers relaxin was detectable in one of every five men or women. It regulates collagen and protects against scar tissue formation. But despite finding it in volunteers, the researchers couldn't directly tie it to joint hypermobility. Relaxin was present, but having it didn't make a person hypermobile.[xxix] In another study they found some connection with joint hypermobility but not in all joints.

What we do know is that relaxin affects many body organs. Women exhibit more relaxin response than men, despite sometimes having lower blood levels: Women had more receptors for relaxin than men did, and didn't need to have as high a blood level to get more effect. In fact, having more relaxin receptors seemed to lower overall blood levels.[xxx]

Some researchers argue that blood levels of the hormone will never reflect true relaxin levels because relaxin is produced in many parts of the body and acts locally rather than entering the bloodstream.[xxxi]

Another hurdle to clarifying if relaxin is indeed the cause of joint hypermobility may be that testosterone offsets the effect of relaxin on ligaments.[xxxii] And aging

41

can blunt the response to relaxin. So by combining both men and women, or women of various ages into a group, no effect of relaxin on EDS will show up. Because the definitive studies haven't been done we cannot currently conclude that relaxin causes EDS, only that it has some yet undefined role in the disease process.

Setting our reservations to the side, let us consider relaxin as a possible Factor X, a possible cause in EDS. If not the syndrome, possibly the pain. Female athletes with higher relaxin levels have four times as much risk of tearing out their knees.[xxxiii] They may not have joint hypermobility, just an increased risk of tearing.

Relaxin meets the criteria for not only affecting the muscles and tissues but also systemically affecting all the body's organs. It not only helps remodel the collagen around all the organs, it also affects basic processes including how fast the body can clot the blood.[xxxiv]

Even as we consider relaxin beyond pregnancy, the very definition of relaxin has changed. Relaxin has been included in the insulin family of hormones. Insulin affects every cell in the body, determining how much sugar is needed. Relaxin has different effects, dilating blood vessels to increase the blood flow to organs and muscles. It also increases the speed of proper healing in every body tissue.[xxxv]

To make things more complicated, we have the discovery of two new kinds of relaxin, called relaxin 2 and relaxin 3. Relaxin 2 works in the body like the original relaxin, but relaxin 3 works directly in the brain. It controls food intake and the stress response, so fluctuation in relaxin 3 levels can increase anxiety.[xxxvi]

In humans relaxin 3 represents uncharted territory. It is an entirely new system of arousal, affecting stress, food, motivation, sleep, and emotional memory.[xxxvii] So, do EDS patients exhibit noticeable changes in these areas? Yes. People with hypermobility have greater levels of fear and more intense fear including panic disorders.[xxxviii]

The increased anxiety of EDS patients can lead them to self-medicate, either with alcohol or food, which again may be in response to changes in relaxin 3 levels in their brains. In rats more relaxin 3 increases both the need for alcohol and the stress response.[xxxix] But it isn't just alcohol that relaxin 3 gets people to crave. In metabolic syndrome patients with poor weight control (overweight, hypertension, sugar imbalances) relaxin 3 levels were much higher.[xl]

While too much relaxin 3 can cause problems in the brain, regular relaxin in the bloodstream may be part of the solution. It can improve blood sugars even on a poor diet. Mice fed fatty food who also got increased relaxin had lower blood sugars than those who just ate the fatty food. Relaxin also decreases the reaction of the body to salt, so it can decrease blood pressure.

Regular relaxin can even stop a heart attack in its tracks. A patient in heart failure who got I.V. relaxin had no symptoms and no side effects.[xli] A brand of relaxin, called Serelaxin, is in trials for heart failure worldwide.

But short of pregnancy or injection of relaxin hormone, how is someone to modify relaxin in the body? Women generate their maximum relaxin during the second half of their menstrual cycle, so for women maximizing their female hormonal balance is the simplest route for maximizing relaxin levels and response. For men, the association with the testes means that balancing male hormones may hold the key to increasing relaxin levels.

The highest level of relaxin in nature can be found in the first breast milk, the colostrum, of animals. Studies of different animals have shown that relaxin can cross-react with different species, though absorption may be an issue. At this point colostrum products do not, to my knowledge, standardize for relaxin levels, and if the pig studies are accurate the levels of relaxin in colostrum drops off within three days of birth.

What about relaxin as a drug? We're in the experimental stages of treatment with a relaxin producing virus, but the treatment is for that "opposite" illness, keloid formation. Currently, pharmacies do not stock relaxin, which is still seen as solely necessary for pregnancy. A determined patient might find it available experimentally, but until it passes the treatment barrier for keloids it is unlikely to be made more widely available as a drug.

While we wait for commercial relaxin to become available, we must explore other possibilities that may be helpful despite not being Factor X.

Hyaluronic acid (HA) has some intriguing aspects, as well as being readily available as an over-the-counter supplement. It stimulates collagen production, and may normalize keloid forming tissues.[xlii] For those with doctors interested in treating EDS, injected HA performed as well as NSAIDS (Advil, Tylenol) for painful joints with fewer side effects.[xliii]

Would taking hyaluronic acid orally do anything? Possibly. It migrates from the body out into the skin tissues, which supports absorption. It didn't build up anywhere in the body, and seemed well tolerated. The body's tissues naturally produce hyaluronic acid and it needs to rebuild that supply every day.[xliv]

But even hyaluronic acid can be difficult to come by as an oral product. Something similar might be glucosamine. We know that this is well absorbed, and available widely. But will something as simple as glucosamine affect EDS? Possibly. People with EDS have a decreased ability to produce their own glucosamine.[xlv] In conjunction to balancing the sex hormones, a trial of something like glucosamine might be useful and relatively inexpensive.

9
WHERE DO WE GO FROM HERE?

Because of the lack of research, we have only ideas and hypotheses so far. While we have no definitive answers, hopefully this short discussion has raised some questions and sparked your interest in finding answers to what may cause the pain for those suffering from EDS and Joint Hypermobility Syndrome beyond genetics and the overuse of joints.

By the time my patients have found me they've exhausted conventional pain medications and are looking for something more than a prescription. Often they have been classified as permanently disabled, so they aren't likely to have the funds or energy to lobby on their own behalf for more research. EDS is largely overlooked because those in pain are usually so concentrated on just getting through the day. They can't picket the statehouse because they can't walk. They can't write their congresswoman because they can't hold a pen or type without agony.

So what can we do? We do what we can with what we have.

In many cases my patients are confused by even what diagnosis to use. Many have been evaluated for mental health, and question whether or not they're "making it up" because their pain seems to vary dramatically from day-to-day. Going through and explaining the systemic and joint aspects of EDS can be very helpful to patients. A few patients have gone on to specialists in EDS, but many work with their primary care prescriber under a now clearly physical diagnosis. Having their entire medical team acknowledging the legitimacy of their pain is a huge first hurdle for many patients.

Along the way to getting daily narcotic pain medication, many patients have been accused of drug seeking behavior by irritated Emergency Room personnel. In defense of the ER doctors, patients with

EDS often show up screaming for pain medications without any visible break or sprain.

Beyond the social stigma and embarrassment they suffer, narcotic usage is a huge issue for patients. They need to wean off narcotics between pain peaks.

The need to wean has nothing to do with trying to get off the drug, it is a preventative measure to lower the patients' tolerance to the narcotic. As a patient's tolerance rises over time, he or she needs larger and larger doses. Eventually the side effects from the medication can force patients to endure less than optimal doses for pain control. So getting a patient's tolerance down by weaning between pain episodes is in everyone's best interest.

For many of my patients the idea of fluctuation in narcotic medication dosage based on pain is a new one. Previously they'd been given a daily dose that had gradually escalated over time as their tolerance mounted. The prescribing doctor may not have trusted that the patient was capable of weaning without hospitalization, so maintained a constant prescription. But I've never met an EDS patient who didn't increase her medication if the pain got too bad, and weaning is the other side of that coin. Since we lack a wide range of proven helpful treatments for EDS, we need to use as little narcotic as we can to prolong its effectiveness.

In my practice patients often learn new ways of moving and walking, sitting and lying down. Many treat pain as a warning sign to remain entirely immobile, as they have been told that using their joints will make it worse. But I have seen better results from patients able to move more. Whether the motion helps the body recover or simply allows the patient greater freedom while dealing with their chronic pain, the most miserable patients I have seen are those who do not move.

Many of the treatments that help ordinary people with muscles aches and strains can have either a helpful or paradoxical effect on EDS patients. The most consistently useful physical support seems to be gentle passive motion and stretching within a normal range of motion. Hard massage will often feel good but can flare a pain episode. Heat is most often helpful, but a cold pack is just the thing at times. Trial and error are necessary parts of any treatment.

While I have not isolated a single environmental factor, many aspects of an EDS person's environment can worsen their condition. The genetic nature of their diagnosis saps both hope and will from many patients, who falsely see their symptomatic elderly relatives as their own preordained fate. So few patients have engaged in their own medical journey, or even been asked to list over the years what made their pain better or worse? Only a few have taken the step of charting their pain, looking for any times of peak pain and trying to figure out what could have set it off. When they do, the reasons for the episode might be anything from job stress to an early menstrual cycle to the start of ragweed season. But looking for a possible cause, avoiding that cause, and seeing decreased pain improves so many aspects of an EDS patient's life.

It is immensely rewarding to have worked with determined, dedicated EDS patients who have improved their relationship with their pain. EDS patients are unbelievable warriors, capable of shrugging off an early morning shoulder dislocation and back tendon tear that would have the rest of us howling in the emergency room. They deserve more attention and time from the medical research community.

ABOUT THE AUTHOR

Christopher Maloney, N.D. is a family doctor who has been blessed with multiple EDS patients. He welcomes reviews of this book on Amazon asking questions, bringing up new research, or asking for better explanations.

His website is: http://maloneymedical.com/ Sign up to receive updates on his newest research.

The endnotes have been modified to provide easy links to the medical research.

[i] Castori M1. Joint hypermobility syndrome (a.k.a. Ehlers-Danlos Syndrome, Hypermobility Type): an updated critique. http://www.ncbi.nlm.nih.gov/pubmed/23407074

[ii] Fransiska Malfait, MD, PhD, Richard Wenstrup, MD, and Anne De Paepe, MD, PhD. Ehlers-Danlos Syndrome, Classic Type Synonyms: Ehlers-Danlos Syndrome, Classical Type; EDS, Classic Type. Includes: Ehlers-Danlos Syndrome Type I, Ehlers-Danlos Syndrome Type II http://www.ncbi.nlm.nih.gov/books/NBK1244/

[iii] http://hypermobility.org/

[iv] Russek LN1, Errico DM. Prevalence, injury rate and, symptom frequency in generalized joint laxity and joint hypermobility syndrome in a "healthy" college population. http://www.ncbi.nlm.nih.gov/pubmed/25930211

[v] Sanches SB1, Oliveira GM, Osório FL, Crippa JA, Martín-Santos R. Hypermobility and joint hypermobility syndrome in Brazilian students and teachers of ballet dance. http://www.ncbi.nlm.nih.gov/pubmed/25218649

[vi] Terry RH1, Palmer ST2, Rimes KA3, Clark CJ4, Simmonds JV5, Horwood JP6. Living with joint hypermobility syndrome: patient experiences of diagnosis, referral and self-care. http://www.ncbi.nlm.nih.gov/pubmed/25911504

[vii]Trinh Hermanns-Lê, Marie-Annick Reginster, Claudine Piérard-Franchimont, et al. Dermal Ultrastructure in Low Beighton Score Members of 17 Families with Hypermobile-Type Ehlers-Danlos Syndrome http://www.hindawi.com/journals/bmri/2012/878107/

[viii] Syx D, Symoens S, Steyaert W, et al. Ehlers-Danlos Syndrome, Hypermobility Type, Is Linked to Chromosome 8p22-8p21.1 in an Extended Belgian Family

[ix] Burcharth J. · Rosenberg J. Gastrointestinal Surgery and Related Complications in Patients with Ehlers-Danlos Syndrome: A Systematic Review http://www.karger.com/Article/Abstract/343738

[x] Juul-Kristensen B1, Kristensen JH, Frausing B, Motor competence and physical activity in 8-year-old school children with generalized joint hypermobility. http://www.ncbi.nlm.nih.gov/pubmed/19822597

[xi] Engelbert RH1, Bank RA, Sakkers RJ, et al, Pediatric generalized joint hypermobility with and without musculoskeletal complaints: a localized or systemic disorder? http://www.ncbi.nlm.nih.gov/pubmed/12612280

[xii] N. Adib, K. Davies, R. Grahame, et al. Joint hypermobility syndrome in childhood. A not so benign multisystem disorder? http://www.ncbi.nlm.nih.gov/pubmed/15728418

[xiii] Castori M1. Joint hypermobility syndrome (a.k.a. Ehlers-Danlos Syndrome, Hypermobility Type): an updated critique. http://www.ncbi.nlm.nih.gov/pubmed/23407074

[xiv] Burcharth J1, Rosenberg J. Gastrointestinal surgery and related complications in patients with Ehlers-Danlos

syndrome: a systematic review.
http://www.karger.com/Article/Abstract/343738

[xv] Chun SG1, Pedro P, Yu M, Takanishi DM. Type IV Ehlers-Danlos Syndrome: A Surgical Emergency? A Case of Massive Retroperitoneal Hemorrhage.
http://www.ncbi.nlm.nih.gov/pmc/articles/PMC3182407/

[xvi] Castori M, Morlino S, Celletti C, et al. Management of pain and fatigue in the joint hypermobility syndrome (a.k.a. Ehlers-Danlos syndrome, hypermobility type): principles and proposal for a multidisciplinary approach.
http://www.ncbi.nlm.nih.gov/pubmed/22786715

[xvii] Agnew P. Evaluation of the child with ligamentous laxity. http://www.ncbi.nlm.nih.gov/pubmed/9030449

[xviii] Rombaut L, Malfait F, De Wandele I, et al. Medication, surgery, and physiotherapy among patients with the hypermobility type of Ehlers-Danlos syndrome.
http://www.ncbi.nlm.nih.gov/pubmed/21636074

[xix] Adib N1, Davies K, Grahame R, et al. Joint hypermobility syndrome in childhood. A not so benign multisystem disorder?
http://www.ncbi.nlm.nih.gov/pubmed/15728418

[xx] Sykes EM Jr. Colon perforation in Ehlers-Danlos syndrome. Report of two cases and review of the literature.
http://www.ncbi.nlm.nih.gov/pubmed/6367507

[xxi] Gąsior-Głogowska M, Komorowska M, Hanuza J, et al. FT-Raman spectroscopic study of human skin subjected to uniaxial stress.
http://www.ncbi.nlm.nih.gov/pubmed/23290820

[xxii] Philip R. Buskohl,1 Michelle L. Sun, et al. Serotonin Potentiates Transforming Growth Factor-beta3 Induced Biomechanical Remodeling in Avian Embryonic Atrioventricular Valves
http://www.ncbi.nlm.nih.gov/pubmed/22880017

[xxiii] Ohno S, Hirano S, Kanemaru S, et al. Transforming growth factor β3 for the prevention of vocal fold scarring.
http://www.ncbi.nlm.nih.gov/pubmed/22252900

[xxiv] Buskohl PR, Sun MJ, Thompson RP, Butcher JT. Serotonin potentiates transforming growth factor-beta3

induced biomechanical remodeling in avian embryonic atrioventricular valves.
http://www.ncbi.nlm.nih.gov/pubmed/22880017

[xxv] Adib N, Davies K, Grahame R, et al. Joint hypermobility syndrome in childhood. A not so benign multisystem disorder?
http://www.ncbi.nlm.nih.gov/pubmed/15728418

[xxvi] Mantle D, Wilkins RM, Preedy V. A novel therapeutic strategy for Ehlers-Danlos syndrome based on nutritional supplements.
http://www.ncbi.nlm.nih.gov/pubmed/15607555

[xxvii] Lamparter S1, Slight SH, Weber KT. Doxycycline and tissue repair in rats.
http://www.ncbi.nlm.nih.gov/pubmed/12032490

[xxviii] Junker JP1, Caterson EJ, Eriksson E. The microenvironment of wound healing.
http://www.ncbi.nlm.nih.gov/pubmed/23321873

[xxix] Wolf JM, Cameron KL, Clifton KB, Owens BD. Serum relaxin levels in young athletic men are comparable with those in women.
http://www.ncbi.nlm.nih.gov/pubmed/23379736

[xxx] Wolf JM, Scher DL, Etchill EW, et al. Relationship of relaxin hormone and thumb carpometacarpal joint arthritis.
http://www.ncbi.nlm.nih.gov/pubmed/23474155

[xxxi] MacLennan AH. The role of the hormone relaxin in human reproduction and pelvic girdle relaxation.
http://www.ncbi.nlm.nih.gov/pubmed/2011710

[xxxii] Dehghan F, Muniandy S, Yusof A, Salleh N.Testosterone reduces knee passive range of motion and expression of relaxin receptor isoforms via 5α-dihydrotestosterone and androgen receptor binding.
http://www.ncbi.nlm.nih.gov/pubmed/24642882

[xxxiii] Dragoo JL, Castillo TN, Braun HJ, et al. Prospective correlation between serum relaxin concentration and anterior cruciate ligament tears among elite collegiate female athletes.
http://www.ncbi.nlm.nih.gov/pubmed/21737831

xxxiv Bani D1, Nistri S, Cinci L, et al. A novel, simple bioactivity assay for relaxin based on inhibition of platelet aggregation.
http://www.ncbi.nlm.nih.gov/pubmed/17572516

xxxv Samuel CS1, Hewitson TD. Relaxin and the progression of kidney disease.
http://www.ncbi.nlm.nih.gov/pubmed/19077683

xxxvi Tanaka M, Furube E, Aoki M, Watanabe Y. Behavioral analysis of relaxin-3 deficient mice.
http://www.ncbi.nlm.nih.gov/pubmed/24640573

xxxvii Smith CM1, Ryan PJ, Hosken IT, et al. Relaxin-3 systems in the brain--the first 10 years.
http://www.ncbi.nlm.nih.gov/pubmed/21693186

xxxviii Smith T, Easton V, Bacon H, et al. The relationship between benign joint hypermobility syndrome and psychological distress: a systematic review and meta-analysis. http://www.ncbi.nlm.nih.gov/pubmed/24080253

xxxix Walker AW1, Smith CM1, Chua BE2, et al. Relaxin-3 receptor (RXFP3) signalling mediates stress-related alcohol preference in mice.
http://www.ncbi.nlm.nih.gov/pubmed/25849482

xl Ghattas MH1, Mehanna ET, Mesbah NM, et al. Relaxin-3 is associated with metabolic syndrome and its component traits in women.
http://www.ncbi.nlm.nih.gov/pubmed/23018057

xli Wilson SS1, Ayaz SI, Levy PD. Relaxin: a novel agent for the treatment of acute heart failure.
http://www.ncbi.nlm.nih.gov/pubmed/25759289

xlii Hoffmann A, Hoing J, Newman A, et al. Role of Hyaluronic Acid Treatment in the Prevention of Keloid Scarring.
http://www.ncbi.nlm.nih.gov/pmc/articles/PMC4054787

xliii Muneaki Ishijima, Toshitaka Nakamura, Katsuji Shimizu, et al. Intra-articular hyaluronic acid injection versus oral non-steroidal anti-inflammatory drug for the treatment of knee osteoarthritis: a multi-center, randomized, open-label, non-inferiority trial
http://www.ncbi.nlm.nih.gov/pmc/articles/PMC3979073/

[xliv] Mariko Oe, Koichi Mitsugi, Wataru Odanaka, Dietary Hyaluronic Acid Migrates into the Skin of Rats
http://www.ncbi.nlm.nih.gov/pmc/articles/PMC4213400/

[xlv] Malfait F, Kariminejad A, Van Damme T, et al. Defective initiation of glycosaminoglycan synthesis due to B3GALT6 mutations causes a pleiotropic Ehlers-Danlos-syndrome-like connective tissue disorder.
http://www.ncbi.nlm.nih.gov/pubmed/23664118

Printed in Great Britain
by Amazon